For Women Over 40

A BIOHACKERS GUIDE TO KETO & FASTING

Rediscover Your Body's Intuition On What And When To Eat

DEBORAH HOLMÉN M.ED, NBCT

Hi! So glad you could join me on this incredible journey!

I was just like you, trying to figure out what had happened to my body once I hit my late 40's. I thought the ravages of stress from teaching for 25 years had finally taken its toll. Stress was only a part of it.

I began to believe I had to accept getting older meant saying goodbye to a young and vibrant body. I loved to cook and followed all of the ADA dietary guidelines, eating the best foods possible, but for some reason, my 5'2" frame was gaining weight rapidly. I was fighting brain fog, fatigue, lack of energy, acne, joint paint, strange rashes, craved carbs and sugars, and watched the scale climb.

I accidentally discovered an old health app on my phone that made me realize the shocking truth; I had gained 25 pounds in less than 18 months, and my doctors were telling me, "You're just getting older."

I share this journey in detail on my blog, "Can You Get Your Body Back After 50? A 4 Part Series on Discovering Your Hurdles, The Science Behind How to Fix Them, and Empowering Your Life!" That's most likely how you found me, and now you are ready to take back what you thought you lost.

In this guide, I will share with you what I learned in the three years of my medical research, uncovering my pitfalls, and the insights I gained to get the life and body back I knew I deserved!

Let's get started!

Debbie Holmén, M.Ed., NBCT, Research Writer

As you read in my blog, "Can You Get Your Life Back After 50?", I shared how the stress from balancing a dynamic teaching career, a new relationship, and writing a screenplay, all contributed to overly stressed Adrenal glands. This gland produces a variety of hormones including adrenaline and the steroids, like cortisol which is released in times of stress. When this system stops working properly, many health-related issues can occur like weight gain, brain fog, fatigue and much more.

Although I began learning in-depth about the adrenal system, I had no idea how much all of my other systems depended on this tiny walnut-sized organ to be at their best.

After much deliberation, I retired from teaching after 25 years to get my health back and dove full-time into my writing career. It was during my research when I realized I had to change my body's fuel. I read hundreds of studies and research on the advancements made in the healthcare industry that questions our dependency on pharmaceuticals and concluded that the Standard American Diet was failing us.

My research led me to various experts in the fields of functional and integrative medicine that taught me how my body was burning the wrong kind of fuel. I could no longer eat the way I used to since it was stressing my body even more. Carbs and sugars, which is found in every processed food, was slowly destroying my body. Spending more time at the gym would only cause more stress on my already stressed adrenal system. Once I learned how fat was a more efficient fuel, I jumped into the Keto way of eating (WOE) and haven't turned back.

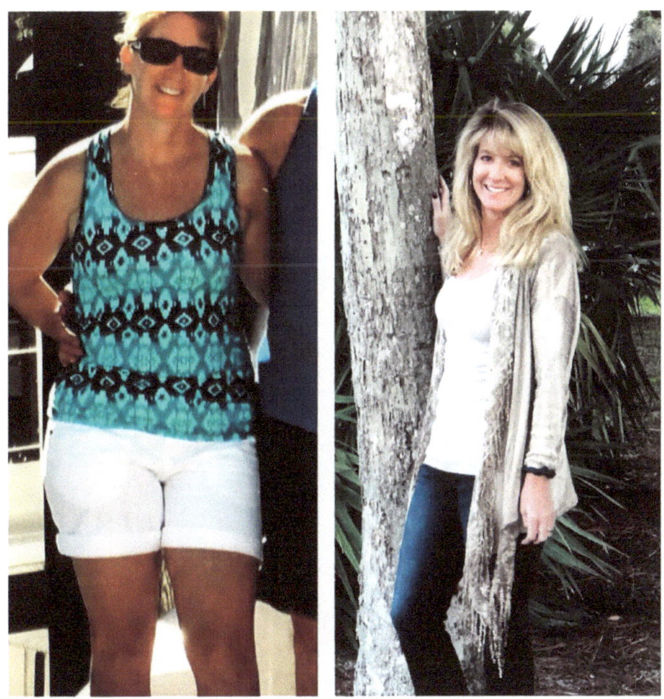

To my surprise, I lost my first 12 pounds in less than six weeks without going to the gym! All of my chronic symptoms went away.

I learned how to create delicious Keto-friendly foods like pizza, popovers, chocolate cake, never missing the sugar-laden forms again. Keto was so satiating since it incorporated more fats, so I felt fuller longer. I noticed I didn't need to eat as often and had more energy and vitality.

CONTENTS

Where To Begin

March 2017, I began researching ways in which women in their 40's were able to regain their health and body back, but most of the websites were about women in their 20's or 30's. Not to exclude our younger sisters, however, a woman in her 40's is dealing with many different issues like the decrease in hormones, changes in careers and family dynamics with children leaving home and aging parents, as well as changes in their marital status. Of course, any of these things can happen to any woman at any age, I wanted to find women that were similar to me.

When I did find websites of women in their 40's, many dealt with their issues by working out for hours on end in Bootcamp-type classes, restricting their calorie intake or paying for specialty foods or weight-loss supplements. None of this felt right for me. I did not need to add additional stressors to my body.

It wasn't until I found, KetoInCanada, a blogger who although was younger shared the same story and my body-type was similar to hers. As I read about her experience, I was jolted back to a time when I did the Atkins diet 18 years ago with much success, however, there were not as many resources back then. Now, there is so much research, as well as amazing Keto recipe bloggers and companies creating foods for the Keto lifestyle.

I waited until April of 2017 to start my Keto lifestyle. We were living on a boat at the time, and I needed better access to grocery stores and pantry storage to make things easier. In May, we moved to Saint Petersburg, Florida where I revamped my pantry. I made sure I knew the carb count of every food I ate, ensuring I was staying between a 20-25 gram carb count every day.

Many Keto Groups suggest women should stay between 20-25 grams of carbs per day due to how our hormones respond to carbohydrates in our system.

I used the My Fitness Pal app to monitor how many carbs I was consuming. I also monitored my blood ketone levels by using Ketone Strips you can purchase at any pharmacy for a nominal cost. These strips let you know approximately what level of ketones you are releasing which helps you choose appropriate low-carb foods.

What Is The Ketogenic Diet?

The Ketogenic diet suggests we eat a total of 70% high-fat, 25% moderate-protein, and 5% low-carbohydrates forcing the body to burn fats rather than carbohydrates.

on the Standard American Diet Guidelines, we should be eating a diet high in fiber and carbohydrates like cereals, grains, pasta, bread, etc. These carbs are then converted into glucose, which in turn fuels our body. We now know that too much glucose is detrimental to our health.

When we reduce our carbohydrate intake, the liver is forced to find a new fuel source to burn. It converts your body's fat into fatty acids and ketone bodies. These ketone bodies pass into the brain and replace glucose as an energy source. Ironically, this fat adapted diet is the brain's preferred fuel of choice, not glucose. Ketones can be monitored through your urine by inexpensive Ketone strips purchased through your pharmacy.

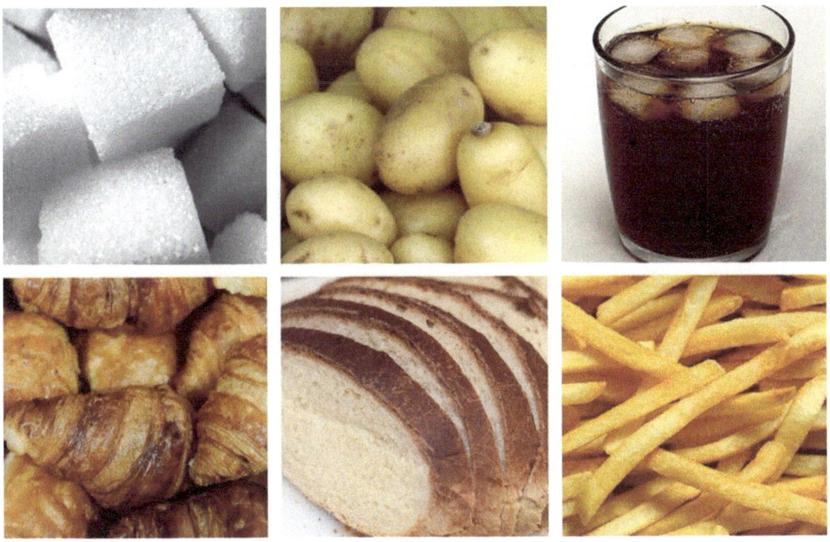

Examples of what we shouldn't be eating. All man-made foods developed by the foods industries. (Except the potato.)

The Ketogenic Diet is also being researched as a diet for healing chronic diseases such as Alzheimer's, diabetes, Parkinson's, and chronic inflammation.

So, now your body is burning its optimal fuel, weight loss becomes inevitable, and healing can begin. This diet is similar to the Paleo and other LCHF diets with the exception that 70% of your food intake should consist of healthy fats, like avocados, grass-fed butter, cream, olive and coconut oils, to name a few. It takes the body about 24-48 hours to deplete all of its stored sugars. When I began Keto, I had headaches and fatigue on the second day detoxing from glucose. I knew once my body switched over to fat burning, these symptoms would cease.

Knowing how to look for carbs and sugars in your food will be the first step, taking the next step will be weaning yourself off of them.

Here's a quick video on how to find out the carbohydrates hidden in your food. Most women should only consume approximately 20-25 carbs per day! This is due to the influence our hormones have in response to food.

How To Count Carbs Video: https://youtu.be/SRC9aCvTPjA

What Are Carbs?

There are three main types of carbohydrate in food:
1) Starches (also known as complex carbohydrates)- all grains, potatoes, pasta, beans, legumes, wheat, barley, quinoa, oats, rice.
2) Sugars- fruit, vegetables, cane sugar.
3) Fiber- the indigestible part of plant foods, including fruits, vegetables, whole grains, nuts, and legumes. When you consume

dietary fiber, most of it passes through the intestines and is not digested.

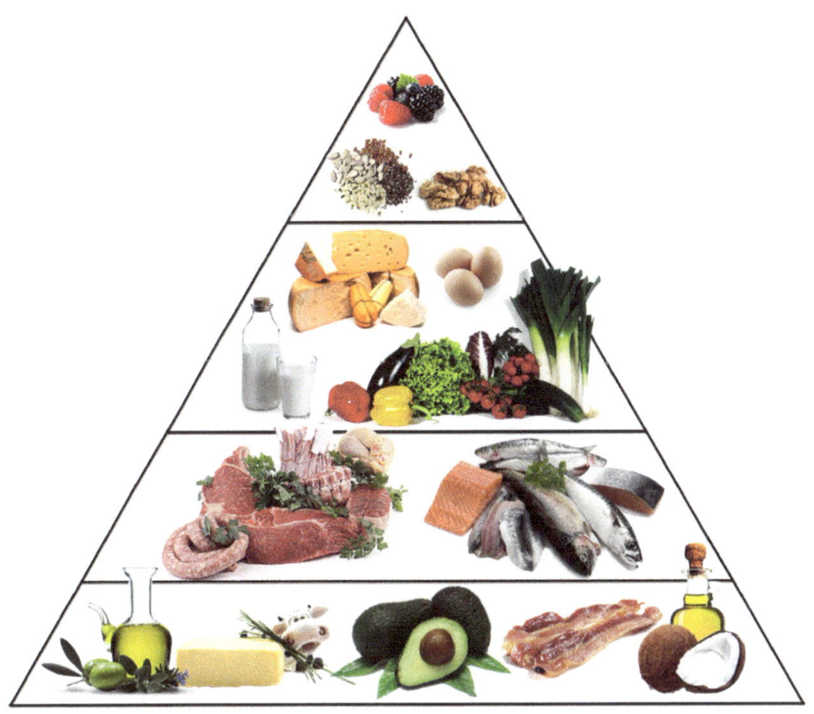

The Ketogenic Diet Food Pyramid

Sugar alcohols are different. These are types of reduced calorie sweeteners produced naturally in plants. Sugar alcohols provide fewer calories than sugar and have less of an effect on blood glucose (blood sugar) than other types of sugar. You can find them in ice cream, cookies, puddings, candies and chewing gum that are labeled as "sugar-free" or "no sugar added."

Examples of beneficial sugar alcohols:

Monk Fruit -granular or drops

Erythritol - Swerve Brand

Xylitol- can cause intestinal discomfort

Stevia- liquid or granular

Even though they are called sugar alcohols, they do not contain alcohol. These healthy low-calorie sweeteners will not negatively impact your gut microbiome like artificial sweeteners do. In addition, these natural sweeteners are useful for reducing carbohydrates when used instead of sugar in coffee, tea, and baking. You can experiment with your own recipes to include low-calorie sweeteners instead of standard sugar or honey.

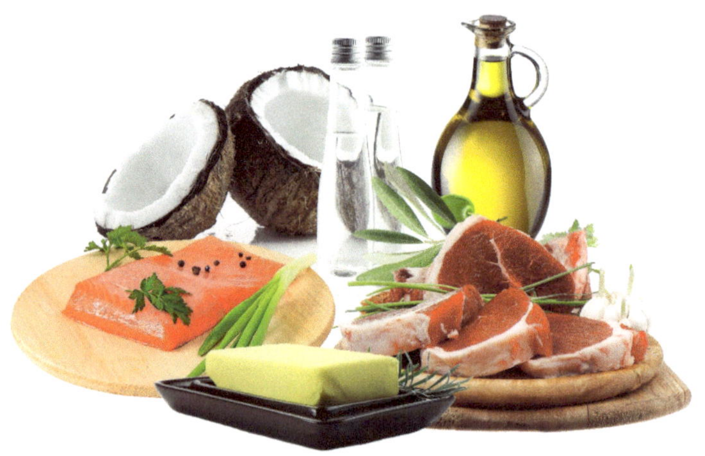

There's a new paradigm shift happening in functional and integrative medicines. Healthy high-fat diets are now replacing the low-fat diets that the ADA thought was best for us in the 1980's. Research is showing 70% of our diet should now consist of foods like avocados, grass-fed butter, and cream, as well as olive and coconut oils, moderate protein and low carbs.

Luckily, I was mentally prepared as my body detoxed from glucose during the first week of ridding myself of carbs. It was the ultimate 'sugar crash' with slight headaches and lightheadedness, but it told me how much I was addicted to sugar. By day 3, my energy and brain clarity was amazing! I could go throughout my day without feeling lightheaded or fatigued. Finally, I was being powered by a high octane fuel; my own fat!

I was disappointed to learn that my doctors didn't really understand LCHF protocols. In fact, they would tell me to go eat a potato as a "power food"! I would crash from the starchy sugars 2 hours later, feeling like I needed to eat again. A vicious cycle for sure! Sugar = quick burn = sugar crash =needing to eat! Not good!

I didn't feel restricted with Keto. If I craved a certain food, I would go online to find a Keto-alternative that was usually better tasting since I could now have real, unadulterated fat. There are now many low carb choices in the stores, which I will share later.

However, Keto wasn't the only change that I had to make that helped me get my body back. Intermittent fasting was the missing link that helped me become totally empowered!

What Is Intermittent Fasting?

This was the game changer for me. Although I had been doing Keto for almost a year, my weight loss stalled after my first five months. I went from 142lbs to 130lbs. I was doing everything a Keto girl should, even counting my Macros, which is noting how much fat, protein, and carbs I was taking in using my health app. This was important because I discovered I was eating too much protein which turns into sugars when your body consumes more than it can burn. I learned I could only eat 6 oz. of protein per day for my 5'2" frame! I used an online Keto Calculator to help me learn my Macros numbers. I lost two more pounds, but it was still not making an impact.

Then while copy editing for Ben Angel's book, UNSTOPPABLE: A 90 Day Plan to Biohack Your Mind and Body for Success, intermittent fasting came into my radar. Out of curiosity, I read several books and watched an incredible documentary about Fasting, The Science of Fasting.

Intermittent Fasting is when you vary eating windows and fasting windows taking advantage of your natural fasting period while you're sleeping for eight hours or more.

The "window" is a period of time you are either fasting or feeding. Typically most fasts last 16 hours to receive the minimum benefits. As an example, you begin your Fasting Window when you finish dinner.

Then the moment you begin eating again, you have broken your fast. This is your eating window.

After I read Dr. Jason Fung's book, The Complete Guide to Fasting, I jumped into a 7-Day Water Fast! (I do not recommend long fasts, unless you are already fat-adapted or eating a low carb diet, and are not on any medications and relatively healthy.)

My 7-Days Fast

I started my fast on March 24, 2018, and didn't eat again until March 31, 2018. I lost the last 12 pounds in that week and felt incredible. Going

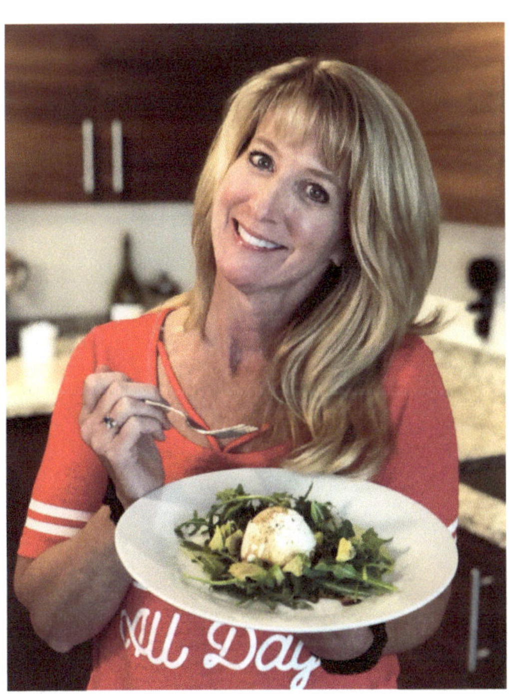

strict low-carb for three days prior helped me cruise through the glucose detox much easier on the second day of fast.

Each day I felt more and more energized. Dr. Fung explains that after fasting 16- 24 hours, you are in complete autophagy; your body is literally cleaning out anything that doesn't belong. Any dysfunctional cells are eaten by the healthy cells that have increased in number due to your new diet, giving you more energy. This energy comes from the newly generated Mitochondria. There is no other way to build more Mitochondria except to fast. After

12 hours of fasting, Human Growth Hormones are also released. HGH is necessary for its anti-aging and longevity effects on the body. So, the longer you fast the better! I was now a believer!

Now I do intermittent fasting to maintain my weight and to keep my insulin under control. One important aspect about fasting is that you have to shake your body up from going into homeostasis and getting used to the same routine, or it will adapt to your way of eating and not be as effective. I have to change my routine often.

How I Do Intermittent Fasting: Everyone Is Different!

On Mondays and Tuesdays, I have a 20-hour fasting window, my eating window opens between 4PM-8PM to allow me to eat with friends and family. I have found my portion sizes have dropped dramatically, so I make sure I eat lots of veggies, healthy fats and lessen my protein. I only drink alcohol occasionally to give my busy liver a break and keep my insulin levels under control.

Then on Wednesday and Thursday, I do an 18 hour fast and 6-hour feeding window. This shakes up my insulin schedule and keeps it out of a routine. Friday I will do another 20:4 to allow for socializing over the weekend and impromptu dinners out. If an event comes up, I just make adjustments.

On the weekends, I go with the flow with my fasting windows and make the best food choices to keep me from having too much glucose in my meals. Keep it easy and fun, and be picky about what you eat! If I overdo it, I know Monday and Tuesday will help me recover.

Fasting is essential for people with chronic illness that want to regain their body's proper functions. There are tons of myths that were created through a lack of knowledge about what fasting does to the body.

We now have hundreds of studies that debunk myths about fasting. Becoming educated with the proper techniques of fasting will help you realize the benefits outweigh any concerns. Links to videos, podcasts and support groups you can join for free are on the Resources Page.

Below is a chart that shows you just a few ways you can embed fasting into your daily life. I started with a Water Fast since I was in the middle of reading Dr. Fung's book. It wasn't until the fourth day of my fast that I incorporated fats into my morning coffee to give me energy. I felt incredible with each day. Hunger really wasn't the issue. It was getting rid of the 'habit' that I had to eat that created the quandary!

Fasting, you will realize, is more of a psychological study of how you relate to food. From the time we are children we grow up with certain beliefs about food and meals. It is the largest social event in our daily lives, so giving up the action of eating yet wanting to be social will bring you through a paradigm shift for sure.

Variations Of Fasting

Variations of Fasting	CLEAN FAST- Water Only	"DIRTY FAST"	FAT FAST
MONDAY A.M. - Typically breakfast is skipped to keep Insulin under control.	Fasting Window- drink only water, tea or plain coffee. No bone broth since that has some proteins that can impact insulin response.	Water, teas coffee, with some fat added to coffee or drink it plain. Add a tablespoon of butter, or coconut oil or MCT oil, or cream.	Bulletproof Coffee - tbs. of Butter, tbs. of coconut oil or MCT oil, Heavy whipping cream. No sweeteners
LUNCH Times can vary to begin eating. Being fat adapted helps you Fast longer.	Break Fast after 16 hours or longer. Eat low carb & good fats. Cheating can lose all of the benefits you've been working so hard toward.	Drink Bone Broth for energy, minerals, and collagen. Bone broth helps sustain longer fasts supporting your body.	Bulletproof Coffee- preferable decaf if you had adrenal issues. Bone broth with a pat of butter. Eat some coconut oil.
DINNER Eating windows should close 3 hours before bedtime.	Examples: 16 Hrs. Fasting: 8 Hrs. Eating OR 17hrs Fast: 7hrs Eat 18hrs Fast: 6hrs Eat 19:5, 20:4, 21:3, etc. Any variation of Fasting/Eating Window = 24 hours	Dirty Fasting allows for more variations during the Fasted state. Fats and bone broth help to keep you energized. Be sure to make good food choices when eating to reap all of the benefits!	20:4 Hour Fast or OMAD One Meal A Day- eating one meal a day can give you variation in what you eat, allowing a less strict diet. Keep sugars & carbs to a minimum for best results.

Benefits of Fasting

Resets Insulin Resistance

Blood levels of insulin drop significantly, which facilitates fat burning, and lowers the risk of Type 2 Diabetes (1). Insulin resistance is corrected.

Increases Human Growth Hormone

HGH works to protect a lean muscle and metabolic balance; a response triggered and accelerated by fasting. During a 24-hour or longer fasting periods, HGH increases an average of 1,300 percent in women and nearly 2,000 percent in men. (2)

Systemic Cellular Repair

The body induces important cellular repair processes called autophagy, such as removing waste material from cells and destroying dysfunctional cells (3). This process begins between the 12th-14th hour of fasting, so fasting for longer than 14 hours greatly enhances the benefits of autophagy as it rids the body of intracellular viruses, bacteria, damaged proteins and subpar organelle creating longevity and strengthens the immune system.

Stimulates Gene Expression

There are beneficial changes in the neurology of the brain stimulating several genes and molecules related to longevity and protection against diseases like Alzheimer's, Parkinson's, and dementia (4, 5).

Aids in Cardiac Health

Fasting drastically reduces LDL- C, "bad cholesterol" and triglycerides, and greatly increases HDL-C, "the good cholesterol"(6)

Saves Money and Time

This was an unexpected benefit during my 7-day long fast. I was able to increase my work productivity and put time toward a walk or yoga since I didn't have to prep for meals or grocery shop.

When you shorten your eating window and feel completely satisfied with wholesome good food, you naturally chose food that tastes great and is good for you. I can have sashimi more often since I'm not spending money on snacks or breakfast ingredients. Great trade-offs for a healthier lifestyle. Bonus!

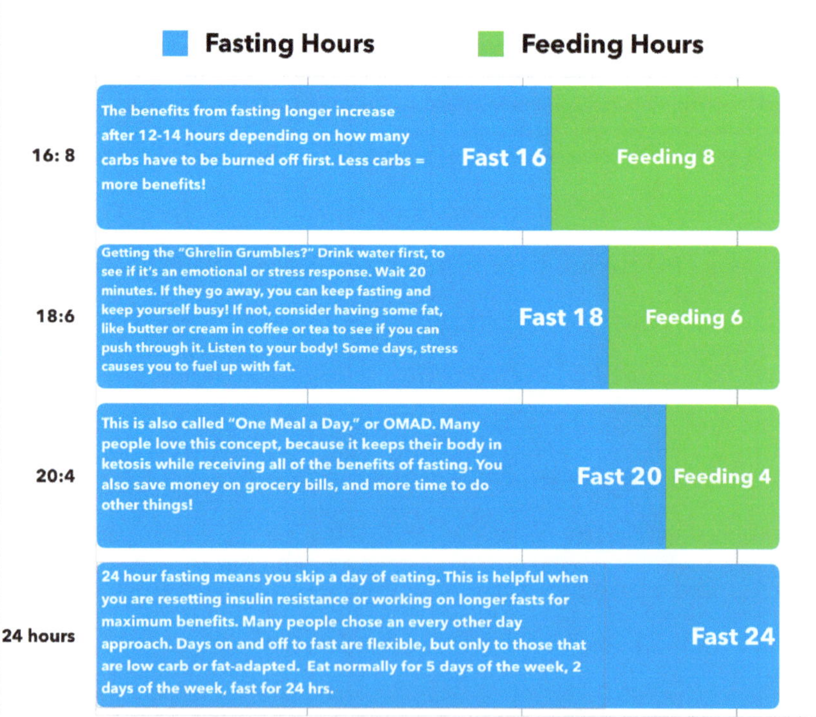

since I'm not spending money on snacks or breakfast ingredients. Great trade-offs for a healthier lifestyle. Bonus!

Fasting: Allow Your Body to Recalibrate

In my blog I share how I first learned of fasting from the French cookbook, French Women Don't Get Fat, by Mireille Guiliano. It was

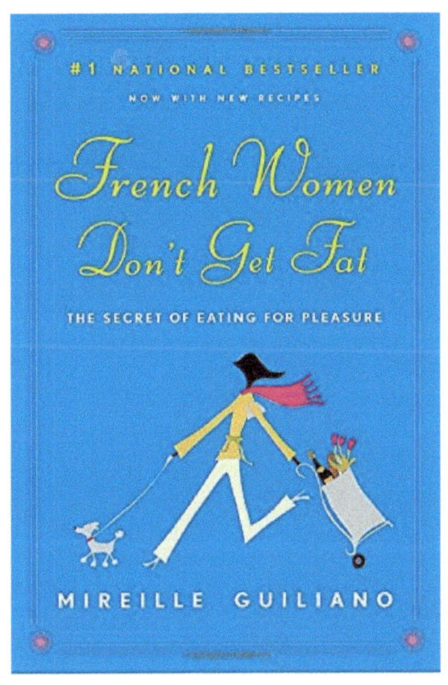

fascinating for me to read that the French art of fasting is passed down from generation to generation to recalibrate the body after times of stress, celebrations and seasons.

She shares how they make a leek-based broth to sip on for three days, and suggests making it a 'retreat' for oneself to get rested and reorganized. The French also teach nutrition in their schools from the primary grades on, so even the children understand eating good food without excess, and to avoid junk food and GMO foods will keep you healthier.

While attending a writers retreat at La Muse in Labastide Esparbairenque, France for three weeks, I was able to watch first-hand how food portions were so much smaller than in America. We have succumbed to the "Supersize" or "Grande" mindset thinking more was better. In France, I followed women down the aisles watching them pick out whole fat creams, cheeses, and yogurts in much smaller packaging. Their aisles of boxed or processed foods are half the size of ours, and their meat and seafood departments were filled with whole foods fresh from local farms.

They also are emphatic about eating within the seasons. The foods available at their peak times have the most nutrients and flavors. France does not allow GMO crops or foods to enter into their agriculture. They also practice proper crop rotation to keep their soil rich in minerals passing the benefits onto the crops that are grown.

If you ever get a chance to eat a potato, tomato or carrot grown in France, you are in for a treat and shock at the same time. The vegetables and fruits grown in France are reminiscent of what our food used to taste like here in America in the 70's. So full of flavor and sustenance, no wonder French cooking is so tasty.

Due to Big Agra and the Food industry in the US taking control of our food sources, we are dealing with quick-growing crops lacking in nutrients and flavor, as well as highly processed foods touted as 'healthy'. It seems fewer and fewer people can remember the taste of a ripe tomato off the vine. I was lucky to have grown up with gardens, and a mother that taught us all how to cook. Ironically, it was mostly French cuisine!

Now it seems we must go back to our roots to rediscover the earth again, and the benefits reaped from growing our own foods.

I am wanting to share some insight as to what happened in America to cause our epidemic of obesity and chronic disease. Ironically, other countries are watching us closely to see how we are dealing with the issues we have created by feeding the masses and allowing monopolies control our way of eating.

Suffering from adrenal fatigue and insulin resistance has shown me how our human bodies rely on good wholesome nutrients, and when we genetically or chemically change our sources of foods, we change our body's natural biomes.

The good news is there is an answer. For me, it was eating a Ketogenic diet and incorporating fasting into my routine. I am still learning about what my body needs. It takes time and listening closely to those nudges of insight as to what it's telling me to do. Sometimes it's to eat and sometimes it's to rest. No matter what, I am having more patience with myself and seeing the results of being kinder and more loving to my body.

Pitfalls, Stalls and Strange Things! Q & A

Keto Flu or Detoxing From Sugar this may occur during the first few days up to a week when beginning the Keto way of eating. This is due to your body detoxing from glucose and other toxins in your system. Once your body begins to burn fat from your food, and stored fat from your body, these symptoms should cease. Burning off your sugar reserves can take from 12 to 48 hours or longer, depending on your health and carb intake. Consuming drinks with electrolytes, or adding extra Himalayan Sea Salt to bone broth helps correct this.

Which Foods Have Carbs? List of Common Foods We Eat With Carb Counts this list is very helpful to get an idea of carbs per serving.

Constipation or The Loosey Goosey's - Constipation can occur when you're dealing with Adrenal Fatigue, as well as when you start Keto or Fasting. Fasting causes your digestive system to go to sleep and rest. By drinking plenty of fluids, you can keep this sleeping giant well hydrated. It's important to eat fiber-laden leafy, green vegetables, but you can also take a fiber supplement to help keep your intestines happy. Natural Calm in Raspberry Lemonade was my go-to drink to help get things moving. You know its working too well when you have to hit the john too often. There are also foods your body might not be accustom to like coconut oil or MCT oils. These can have a laxative effect, so starting with smaller amounts may help. You also may be suffering from Increased Intestinal Permeability (IIP medical term, or "Leaky Gut") This is when your gut flora is out of whack. Too much "bad bacteria" kills off your good bacteria, so you will experience symptoms of discomfort. See "Probiotics."

What is Adrenal Fatigue? How do I know if I have it? Adrenal fatigue occurs when we are in constant fight or flight response mode. Chronic stressors cause our adrenals to overwork and are no longer providing our bodies with the proper adrenal response, instead it pumps out too much Cortisol, the stress hormone.

Cortisol causes weight gain as visceral fat in the midsection. Dr. Berg has a great webinar that shows you the Adrenal Body types to help you decide if you have this syndrome. 85% of most women do! Take Dr. Berg's Free Body Type Quiz to see what could be the cause of your symptoms.

What is Insulin Resistance? How do you fix your Insulin? Insulin is a hormone that facilitates the transport of blood sugar (glucose) from the bloodstream into cells throughout the body for use as fuel. When we eat, the pancreas secretes insulin into the bloodstream. With insulin resistance, the normal amount of insulin emitted is not sufficient to move glucose into the cells – thus the cells are said to be "resistant" to the action of insulin. To compensate, the pancreas secretes insulin in larger amounts to maintain adequate blood-sugar movement into cells and keep normal blood sugar levels. This is potentially the start of pre-diabetes. To reverse this effect, you need to turn off your insulin response for long periods of time through fasting and not eating. A 16 to 18-hour fasting window or longer, as well as eating a low carb low sugar diet, will help reset insulin resistance so your body becomes insulin sensitive again. Visit Dr. Jason Fung on Youtube for more info.

Should I take supplements? This will be different for everyone, especially for those that are needing to heal from a chronic disease. I recommend you find a Functional or Integrative Medicine doctor in your area to go over your specific needs.

Which supplements help in Keto or Fasting regimens? I knew I needed to support my body with high quality essential fatty acids, as well as Vitamins that my body would not be getting due to the quality of food that is now grown in the United States. Since the 1970's the quality of our soils, have decreased tremendously. The spinach your grandmother ate provided her with the necessary minerals needed for her body. Now, we have to eat approximately 8 pounds of spinach to get the same amount of trace minerals. I take Omega 3's, MCT oil, Vitamin D, B-Complex vitamins for stress, as well as several forms of Magnesium for mental clarity and focus. I also cycle my supplements by taking the necessary dosage for a month or two, then stop for a week. This way I can see how I'm doing and adjust dosages. You will need to experiment with what your body needs. Trust your instincts and your gut!

Do I have to eat Keto? I am more of a vegetarian. - The beauty of fasting is that you are still regulating how your body deals with lowering its insulin response. Keeping yourself away from processed foods is critical, so your body can quickly burn any stored glucose and start burning fat. It is suggested that vegetarians need to up their intake of fats like coconut oils, avocados, etc., to keep their body well fueled. Finding alternatives to pasta and carbs is beneficial. Read this quick article on what to eat and avoid if you are a vegetarian.

Can I eat a regular diet if I fast? Most healthy people, with no chronic illnesses, can eat a regular diet and still benefit from fasting. However, they usually have to fast for longer hours to burn off glucose. It is still important to keep processed sugars to a minimum for overall wellbeing.

What is the shortest amount of time can I fast? The longer the fast, the more benefits you receive. Typically a 16-hour fasting window starts the anti-aging effects of HGH being released into the body, as well as autophagy and cellular replacement. These essential anti-aging processes don't begin until around the 12th hour and continue while fasting, so stopping a fast shortly after the 12th hour reduces the benefits. For people with Insulin resistance, Dr. Jason Fung states an 18-hour fasting window or longer helps to reset the insulin resistance.

What if I cheat? Was it for emotional reasons? Were you craving a certain food? Were you stressed or bored? There are so many reasons why people cheat, and it will take some sleuthing to discover the reason. Sometimes the body craves something that's deficient, like iron or minerals. Something stressful could have also triggered your "hunger hormone" ghrelin. Ghrelin is released in times of stress, so drink water to calm the grumbles, before going for a box of snacks. The good news is you can always start over, but be mindful as to the reasons why you're cheating.

During my 7-day fast, I was astonished as to how much of a habit eating was for me. When 10 AM and 2 PM rolled around, I wanted to snack. I wasn't really hungry per se; it was just a habit I developed when I was a teacher. Those were the two times in the day I could grab a snack. This 25-year-old habit I had to stop. To break these habits, I now stop and think, "Why am I hungry?" Then, I make a cup of tea or drink warm water with a dropper full of Licorice Root or cinnamon since both reduce blood glucose levels.

Many times the reason we feel hungry is due to our insulin levels increasing since we had too many carbs the day before. We have to burn off the excess glucose before our body uses our own stored fat for energy.

Is it painful to fast? I'm nervous about how hungry I'll be. I was surprised at how the hunger pangs were not that bad; like typical hunger without the hypoglycemic drops. Since the 1980's we've been led to believe that we should keep hunger at bay, to snack throughout the day to keep your metabolism from slowing down. However, none of these concepts were based on scientific research. Many studies were financed by the food industries to promote their products, thus making us believe we had to eat six times a day. You all remember hearing that sugar wouldn't cause heart disease and low-fat diets were safe. Sadly, we believed the hype. Allowing your body to reset its hunger signals helps us understand what we really need. I learned so much about what hunger feels like versus being bored or needing comfort. Keeping busy during fasting hours really helps the time pass. Journaling your thoughts during times of hunger also helps us understand our relationship with food again.

Is Keto my only choice for a way of eating? No, it's not! Exciting, right? But you have to be mindful if you're eating real food or not. I hear people saying they're living a Keto lifestyle then eat high-carb foods. If they are still getting the results without complaint or illness, then they are the lucky ones. However, studies have shown that getting rid of processed foods, sugars and simple carbs are in their best interest to keep them from developing chronic disease. Dave Asprey, the founder of Bulletproof Coffee, put millions of dollars into getting his health back. So, let his research and efforts help you with his free guide to various ways of eating. Play around with various foods and see if you like the results. Your gut will tell you or not! Free Bulletproof Diet Roadmap

The Four Aspects of You

In Part 4 of my series, "Can You Get Your Body Back After 50?" I share how I had to look inward before looking outward. I wrote down anything and everything that seemed to be amiss in my life. I couldn't blame this on anyone, except me. It was "how I was reacting" to life that was making me sick. I knew I could no longer control what happened to me in life, but I could surely change how I reacted to it.

The body demonstrates 'dis-ease' by giving warning signals; headaches, joint aches, stomach issues, weight gain, skin eruptions, etc. If these "warnings" go unchecked, it can develop into something more chronic; inflammation, irritable bowels, food sensitivities, diabetes, migraines, weight gain, ovarian cysts, heart issues, thyroid issues, and the list goes on.

Only a mere 4% of the American population are born with a genetic disease, so we have to look closer at the onset of illness as a psychosomatic response from within our environment and our body. Modern medicine in the United States, although revolutionary in its technology and sciences, is not efficiently making this science readily available to the average citizen due to bureaucratic financial strain, as well as lack of a sustainable delivery system. We have to become our own 'biohacker.'

You already know the answers to your issues, but addressing them will be the most difficult step.

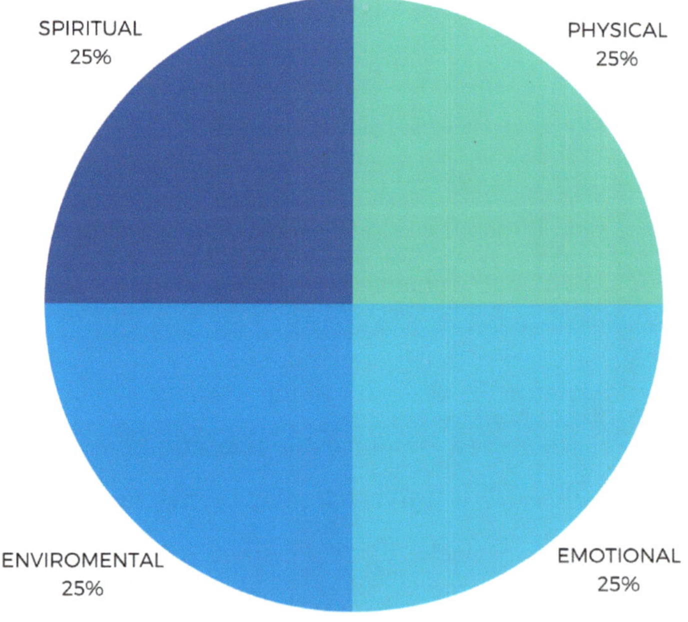

Writing down the 4 areas in your life that you react to on a daily basis helps you decipher what changes need to be made.

- Do we need to look closer at the friends we keep?

- Do they hold us in high-esteem, and help us be the best we can be, or do they enable you, allowing you to repeat negative patterns?

- Is your job fulfilling?

- How do you react with your co-workers?

- Do you feel that everything that goes wrong at work is someone else's fault, or could it be how you are reacting to those things that go wrong?

- Do you honor your body and take care of it?

- Are times with family members detrimental to your health and wellbeing?

These are hefty questions you need to look at closely, then make the necessary changes. Your decisions will not be selfish or rude. They are for your betterment. You will realize this may be the first time in your life you took care of yourself first.

Become empowered!

Take the Holmes & Rahe Stress Scale Test to see if the stressors in your life will lead to illness if they aren't dealt with properly. It's important to make changes in the areas that are causing you too much stress. Ignoring it will only cause your body to react in a negative way. Most likely, your body will start to show the signs of possible chronic ailments, which you won't be able to ignore it any longer.

The good news is that stress is reversible, and chronic diseases are also curable! Finding a Functional or Integrative medicine clinic would be a great first step.

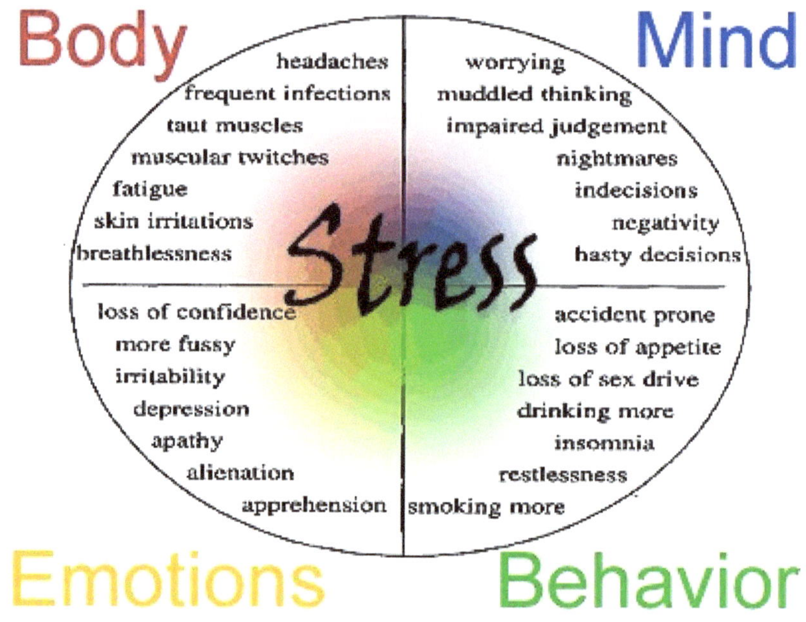

Biotechnology and Tests For Our Health & Wellbeing

While copyediting Ben Angel's book, I was able to try out various biotechnology devices Ben was using to help him biohack his health. The most impressive device is the TouchPointsTM. These devices are attached to your wrists like watches and work by using Bilateral Alternating Stimulation Tactile technology. It softly buzzes disrupting the negative loop in the brain. Tests have proven that stress is reduced

74% in just 30 seconds of use! We were blown away. I tried the devices multiple times when I was feeling stressed. Ben would try to bring my stress levels up by talking about the stressors, but I literally could not stay angry. I couldn't even pose a negative thought and was able to rationally discuss the issues.

The research on the benefits of TouchPoints on cortisol levels, pain, performance, attention, sleep, irritability, and quality of life is astounding. Currently, the company is successfully using these devices for children with Autism, Veterans with PTSD, as well as schools.

Read the Science behind these amazing devices!

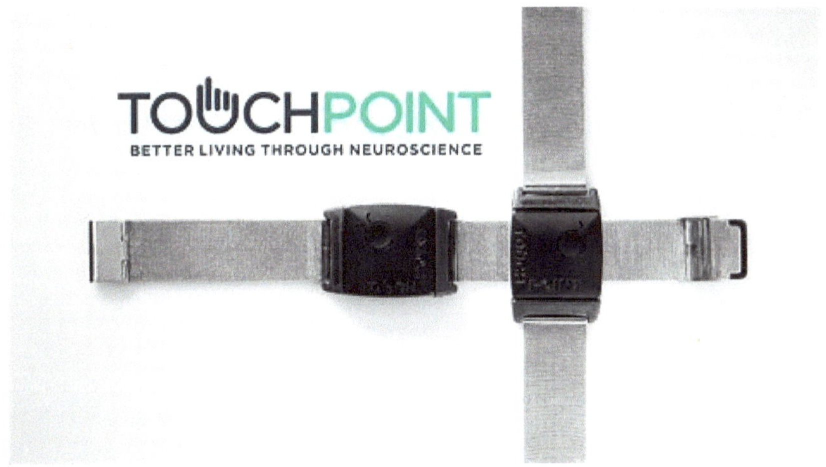

Probiotics and Testing Your Gut Microbiome

I could write a complete guide on these little critters, however, what we are learning about our gut microbiome is changing how we are approaching human health and disease.

These bacteria are essential for maintaining our overall health and wellbeing by producing several vitamins we do not have the genes to make. They also break down our food to extract nutrients we need to survive and teach our immune systems how to recognize dangerous invaders. These helpful bacteria produce anti-inflammatory compounds that fight off other disease-causing microbes.

An ever-growing number of studies have demonstrated that changes in the composition of our microbiomes correlate with numerous diseases, raising the possibility that manipulation of these communities could be used to treat disease.

New studies demonstrate how 'good' bacteria keeps the body metabolically fit, and how an imbalance can cause ill-health effects. Scientists are also learning that we can literally impact our microbiome within hours of eating the good bacteria, contrary to what they used to believe.

Just recall a time you ate some food and within the hour, if not within minutes, your body uncomfortably expelled it! It was your gut microbiome at work!

Ben shares in his book how he had his gut microbiome tested by Thryve, a company offering at-home tests for people who want to see what's impacting their health.

The company sends you a Gut Microbiome Testing Kit. Then the company analyses a stool sample that you provide, and they create a personalized probiotic for you to reintroduce the missing bacteria your gut needs to thrive. What was interesting when Ben received his results, was that he had an enormous amount of bacteria that caused his body to expel invaders. He often had diarrhea after eating which explained the presence of this bacteria. Once Ben started taking his personalized Probiotic formula, he became regular within a day!

Research organizations that are studying Inflammatory Bowel Disease, Colitis, Celiac and Crohn's disease are looking to the NIH's Human Microbiome Project to provide answers to curing these chronic diseases through creating a healthy microbiome.

So what can you do? Getting a personalized test is your best bet, as well as introducing a high-quality probiotic that is shelf-stable is number one.

According to studies, our bodies need to have over 13 strains of probiotics to receive the correct balance of good bacteria since most will die in our stomach acids before reaching their home in the intestines and colon.

Also, don't rely on the ones in the common grocery store to be shelf-stable. Many bacteria die in transit. That's why I chose Garden of Life Probiotics. The probiotic formulas have been well researched and scientifically created by David Perlmutter, M.D. He is an expert in the study of the human microbiome, a board-certified neurologist, Fellow of the American College of Nutrition, America's brain-health expert and #1 New York Times best-selling author of the book, The Grain Brain.

Sugar is also the leading cause of healthy bacteria die-out in our gut. When we ingest too much sugar, we kill off our good bacteria causing multiple symptoms. Candida, as an example, is a beneficial fungus that helps with digestion. However, when too much sugar is consumed, candida can overpopulate since its energy source is glucose. Too much of one type of bacteria causes an imbalance in the whole system. Stop eating sugar, and the excess candida dies off.

The signs and symptoms of Candida can include UTI's, coated tongue, "Candida breath," fatigue, brain fog, digestive issues, sinus infections, recurring yeast infections, mild depression, joint pain, and much more.

The Candida Diet website is a great resource if you're suspecting an overgrowth of Candida, which could be the culprit. But one thing is for sure, SUGAR is the nemesis in most chronic diseases and getting rid of it in our diet is crucial.

Begin Your Path to Rediscovering the Body You Once Had.

The beauty of having this new knowledge of fasting and eating a lower carb diet is that you can make it your own. If you embrace this new way of eating, you will learn the foods and stressors that trigger your weight gain. If you get side-tracked by celebrations or family constraints, you can go right back and reset your body. When you feel hungry, remember to drink water and evaluate why you're hungry before breaking those hard-earned fasting benefits.

Keto Way Of Eating (WOE) - You should take 1-2 Weeks to switch your body from a carb burner to a Fat Burner. Depending on your health, it's necessary to reduce carbs and eliminate sugar from your diet. ***People with Chronic Illnesses diagnosed by their doctor should work with their doctor on monitoring their prescribed medications. Most Type 2 Diabetics can potentially reduce their insulin intake when committing to this WOE, so it will be crucial for you to have regular tests. Please check with your physician before beginning any dietary changes. Most Functional and Integrative doctors are well versed in Keto and Fasting techniques.***

Fasting - I recommend using inexpensive Ketone Strips you can purchase from your pharmacy. These pee-strips will tell you your level of ketones in your urine helping you decide if you need to cut back on your carbs during your Eating Window. Once you are fat adapted, you can begin your fasting protocol. Start with a 16-hour fasting window and an 8-hour eating window. Once you feel an increase in energy, you can increase your Fasting window. This is your body telling you that you are now burning YOUR FAT reserves and turning it into high-octane fuel.

Vary your fasting windows each week, so your body doesn't become accustomed to fasting. Mix it up! Make your fasting work with your schedule and socializing. This is when you'll begin to gain control of your body again and feel the most empowered!

Check your health markers! Re-evaluate how you're feeling, sleeping, as well as how you're doing emotionally and spiritually. Tweaking things through trial and error will help you gain more insight on how your body handles various factors.

Where Should I Begin?

Do You Suffer from A Chronic Illness and on Medication ***Please work with your Functional or Integrative Medical doctor before starting Keto ***

Keep a food journal for the first week or two. I used the MyFitness Pal App to monitor my foods, weight, and carbs intake. This app will show you where carbs can hide!

Food sensitivity Depending on your food sensitivities, a Gut Microbiome test can reveal which foods may be causing your symptoms. You may be able to bring back certain foods once your immune system and gut microbiome is restored.

Cut out all processed sugars and carbs. You can find alternative recipes via Keto Cooking websites.

Listen to Intermittent Fasting and Keto Podcasts to educate yourself on how your body works, pay attention to cravings. You'll get some great feedback on ways to get through stalls.

For Weight Loss with NO Chronic Illnesses - Take 1- 2 weeks to lower your carb and sugar intake. Drink a lot of water during this period. Keep track of your energy levels, stomach issues, and overall wellbeing. You should notice a significant difference within the first week.

BEFORE you go out to dinner, check out the menu online. Most restaurants are great at swapping out chips with crudités or lettuce for hamburger buns.

Online support groups are a great place to find like-minded people getting their health and life back like my Facebook Group, The Biohackers Space Group Facebook has many Keto and Fasting support groups that can help with questions, recipe ideas, and support.

Bring keto snacks and stevia when you travel or go out with friends to tweak drinks and coffee. Ask for cream instead of half-n-half or milk. Wear ankle and wrist weights while cleaning or walking to trick your body into burning more!

Keep a self-care journal on how you're honoring yourself with positive friends, positive activities, and positive affirming words.

Videos For Keto & Fasting

Knowledge is Power!

- Keto for Obesity, Diabetes and Metabolic Syndrome by Dr. Westlake, Duke University

- Therapeutic Fasting with Dr. Jason Fung

- Why French Women are Healthy & Can Eat Everything by Justine Leconte

Resources, Websites, Podcasts & Recipes

Functional/Integrative Doctors and Nutritionists ONLINE

Dr. Mercola

Dy Ann Parham

Dr. Jason Fung

Dr. Eric Westman

Dr. Josh Axe

Dr. David Perlmutter

Dr. Steven Gundry

Dr. Dominic D'Agostino

Podcasts in iTunes and Youtube

Intermittent Fasting Podcast

Dr. Berg Healthy Keto & Intermittent Fasting

The Obesity Code Podcast

Recipes

Keto Recipes - My Favorite   - Pinterest Key Words- "Keto," "Fasting"

Queen Keto

Inspirational People to Follow on Facebook or Instagram

I Am Keto in Canada

Justine Leconte- Officiel!

Keto Transformations on Instagram

Maria Mind Body Health Keto Karma

The Diet Doctor

Keto Karma

Ditch The Carbs

I Breathe, I'm Hungry

Maria, Mind, Body

Keto Pantry Overhaul Food List

VEGETABLES

Artichoke	Brussels Sprouts
Arugula	Cabbage
Asparagus	Carrots
Avocados	Celery
Beets/Beet Greens	Collards
Bell Peppers	Cucumbers
Bok Choy	Eggplant
Broccoli	Garlic
Broccoli Rabe	Green Beans
	Jerusalem Artichoke

Kale
Mushrooms
Olives
Onions
Parsnip
Peppers (all kinds)
Pumpkin
Radish
Romaine Lettuce
Sea Vegetables
Spinach
Squash
Tomatoes
Turnip Greens
Watercress
Wheat Grass
In Moderation:
Brown/Wild Rice
Beans
Sweet Potato
Quinoa

MEAT

(Organic, grass-fed)Beef Bison
Chicken
Duck
Eggs
Lamb
Turkey
Quail, other wild game Venison,
other wild game NO Pork

FISH

(Wild Caught only, NO Farm
Raised) Anchovies
Bass
Cod
Grouper
Haddock
Halibut

Herring
Mackerel
Mahi Mahi
Red Snapper
Salmon
Sardines
Seabass
Trout
Tuna
Walleye
7 NO Shellfish

DAIRY

(Raw, or Low-Temp Processed)
A2 Cows Milk
A2 Cows Cheese
A2 Cows Amasai
Goats Milk
Goats Cheese
Kefir (Cultured Goat Milk)
Sheep Cheese
Sheep Yogurt
Any Other Raw Dairy

NUTS AND SEEDS

Almonds
Brazil Nuts
Chia Seeds
Flax Seeds
Hemp Seeds
Hazelnuts
Macadamia
Pecans
Pine Nuts
Pistachios
Pumpkin Seeds Sesame Seeds
Walnuts
Nut Butters
Seed Butters
NO Peanuts

FATS /OILS

(Organic Unrefined) Avocado Oil
Almond Oil
Butter (pastured) Coconut Oil/Milk Ghee
Grapeseed Oil
Macadamia Oil
Olive Oil
Sesame Oil
Palm Oil
Walnut Oil
NO Canola Oil

SPICES AND HERBS

Basil
Black Pepper
Cayenne Pepper Chili Pepper
Cilantro
Coriander Seeds Cinnamon
Cloves
Cumin
Dill
Fennel
Garlic
Ginger
Mint
Mustard Seeds Nutmeg
Oregano
Paprika
Parsley
Peppermint Rosemary
Sage
Tarragon
Thyme
Turmeric

FRUITS Preferred

Blackberries
Blueberries
Cranberries
Goji Berries
Raspberries
Strawberries
FRUITS In Moderation African
Mango
Apple
Apricot
Banana
Cantaloupe
Camu-Camu
Cherries
Coconuts
Figs
Grapefruit
Grapes
Indian Gooseberry Lemon
Lime
Mango
Nectarine
Orange
Papaya
Peaches
Pears
Pineapple
Plums
Pomegranate Rhubarb
Watermelon All other fruits

CONDIMENTS

Apple Cider Vinegar
Balsamic Vinegar
Coconut Vinegar
Coconut Aminos
Cocoa
Extracts (e.g., Vanilla/Almond)
Guacamole
Hummus

Mustard (Stone Ground) Mayo
(Grapeseed Oil)
Salsa
Sea Salt
Tamari

BEVERAGES
Almond Milk
Coconut Kefir
Coconut Milk
Cultured Whey
Herbal Teas
Kombucha
Raw Vegetable Juices
Sparkling Water
Spring Water (or Filtered)

SWEETENERS
In Moderation

Raw Honey
Stevia
Monk Fruit sweetener

OCCASIONAL INDULGENCES
Wine
DarkChocolate

SUPPLEMENTS
Magnesium
Vitamin D3
Potassium
Shelf-Stable Probiotics
Prebiotic fibers- glucomannan, psyllium husk, konjac root
Super Greens Powder
Whole Food-Based Vitamins
Omega-3 Fish Oil